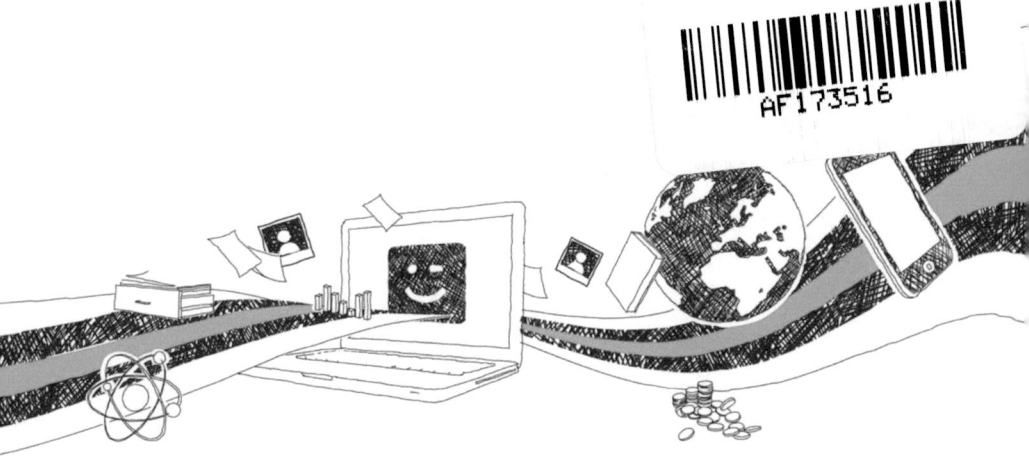
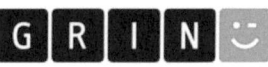

Nora Demattio

HIV/AIDS in Latin America - The Feminization of HIV/AIDS

Gender, Power and its Implications concerning the Epidemic

GRIN Publishing

Bibliographic information published by the German National Library:

The German National Library lists this publication in the National Bibliography; detailed bibliographic data are available on the Internet at http://dnb.dnb.de .

Imprint:

Copyright © 2009 GRIN Verlag, Open Publishing GmbH
Print and binding: Books on Demand GmbH, Norderstedt Germany
ISBN: 978-3-656-10846-7

This book at GRIN:

http://www.grin.com/en/e-book/187459/hiv-aids-in-latin-america-the-feminization-of-hiv-aids

GRIN - Your knowledge has value

Since its foundation in 1998, GRIN has specialized in publishing academic texts by students, college teachers and other academics as e-book and printed book. The website www.grin.com is an ideal platform for presenting term papers, final papers, scientific essays, dissertations and specialist books.

Visit us on the internet:

http://www.grin.com/

http://www.facebook.com/grincom

http://www.twitter.com/grin_com

HIV/AIDS in Latin America - The Feminization of HIV/AIDS

Gender, Power and its Implications concerning the Epidemic

University Vienna

2008

Name: Nora Demattio

Table of Contents

1. Introduction 3

2. Women and HIV/AIDS in Latin America...3

3. *Machismo* and *Marianismo* – Gender Constructions in Latin America 4

    3.1 *Machismo*...4

    3.2 *Marianismo*...5

    3.3 Implications for Women and for Programs and Organsisations

    concerning HIV/AIDS...6

4. Conclusio 9

References 11

1. Introduction

Around the world, in the last decades since the appearing of HIV/AIDS, the prevalence of women infected by HIV is raising faster than the prevalence of men. Although this development had been recognized soon, it was not posible to stop it.

On the basis of these facts, I will have a closer look at the situation of women in Latin America concerning the disease and Iwant to review the "feminization" of HIV/AIDS.

Furthermore, I will give an overview of two Gender constructing concepts of Latin America, *Machismo* and *Marianismo*, which I seek to challenge in its impacts on (the development of) programs and organsisations concerning the epidemic, and following, in women.

2. Women and HIV/AIDS in Latin America

UNAIDS announced in its AIDS Epidemic Update 2007, that the proportions of women living with HIV in Latin America is steadily growing. (UNAIDS 2007: 3)

The estimated number of people living with HIV in Latin America has been 1.400.000 in 2001 and 1.700.000 in 2007, which remains relatively stable at about 0.5%. Nevertheless, while in 2001 about 450.000 of female population (15+) had been infected, in 2007 the number was already at 550.000, which is an increase of the epidemic in women from 32.1% to 32.4%. Although it doesn`t seem to be much at first sight, this probably results in the dramatically growth of infected children (0-14), from 36.000 in 2001 to 44.000 in 2007, which means an increase of about more than 20%. (UNAIDS 2008a: 230f)

According to UNAIDS, the main reason for this development is the transmission of the virus by men - who are likely to have been infected through injecting drug use, or during unprotected paid sex or sex with other men - to the female partners. Futhermore, the transmission in Latin America is primarily seen to "occur among populations at higher risk of exposure". (UNAIDS 2007: 31) This implicates an inner contradiction for me, as exposure demands a degree of posibility to reject from it, which is in many cases not always feasible.

In the literature transmission is refered to activity or, as one can see, mostly to men and their risk-behaviour, which seems quite plausible. In contrary, prevention and prevention programs focus mostly on "vulnerable" groups, which somehow nearly always allude to women, and high-risk groups like *Injecting Drug Users* (IDUs), *Men who have Sex with Men* (MSM) and *Female Sex Workers* (FSWs). (UNAIDS 2008a:213)

This appears to me partly as an obstacle to decrease the prevalence of HIV/AIDS, as in this way one of the main reasons of the spreading of the disease happens to be somehow excluded: the hetero and/or (hidden) bisexual man.

So, consequential, for me talking about the "feminization" of HIV/AIDS in Latin America should also include talking about and reflecting Gender, as well as Gender constructions and concepts in and of Latin America, especially concerning programs to decrease the prevalence of the epidemic.

3. *Machismo* and *Marianismo* – Gender Constructions in Latin America

On the Basis of the feminist groundswell around the 1970s - during the early research on Gender in Latin America, conducted on, by an for women - two concepts gained popularity in the scientific world: *Machismo* and its "counterpart" or compensatory complex *Marianismo*. (Chant 2003: 6ff)

In this chapter I seek to give an overview of these two concepts. I will further analyse possible implications deriving from them, on programs and organisations concerning HIV/AIDS, and following on womens health.

3.1 *Machismo*

„If there is one term which is unambiguously associated with Latin America, it is the term *macho*, and its derivates *machismo* and *machista*." (Melhuus/Stolen 1996: 14)

Machismo is seen as the epitome of (exaggerated) masculinity, which is conceived as something that men are not born with, but must constantly earn. Among the characterisation of the term *Machismo*, the basic tenor lies in the conviction of power and control over women, as well as over other men. (Chant 2003: 14)

Nevertheless, in early works on Gender in Latin America in the 1970s and 1980s, the focus had been on its impact on women, emphasizing the beliefs in male primacy, in man's rights to control women, as well as in male strength and (sexual) potency. This was seen as contributing to a polarisation of Gender roles and as providing cultural legitimation for abuse of women. Furthermore, men, or more precisely *Machos*, had been described as "irresponsible husband" and "distant father", which is a picture that has been soon obsolete. (Chant 2003: 14f)

Work on men has helped to deconstruct some of the stereotypes which were associating men with power and women with powerlessness, but it is to mention that stereoptypes usually do have some ground in practice. Male domination and/or mistreatmentof women is evident, as well as the reference of particular modes of behaviour to *Machismo*, by both man and women. (Chant 2003: 14 and 16)

3.2 *Marianismo*

"Among the characteristics of this ideal are semidivinity, moral superiority, and spiritual strength. This spiritual strength engender abnegation, that is infinite capacity for humility and sacrifice." (Stevens 1973: 94)

The appearance of *Marianismo* in the Gender literature is normally associated with Evelyn Stevens. (Zuckerhut 2008) It is seen as emerged during the colonialism in Latin America, through the influence of the Catholic Church, and has its roots in the worship of the Virgin Mary.

Marianismo stands for idealized femininity, which emphasises the spiritual and moral superiority to men. This again was used, stated Stevens (1973: 94), and contributed to legitimate the subordinate domestic and societal role of women.

Marianismo implicates for them also the "obligation" to remain sexually pure and abstain from sexual activity - in contrary to *Machismo* for the male population - unless for becoming pregnant, although she should also be submissive to the demands of the men. As their connection with childbirth, a "unique opportunity to fulfill God`s will", was perceived to bridge the natural and supernatural worlds, women receive a higher status in the if they have children and are caring mothers. (Chant 2003: 10; Stevens 1973: 94; Zuckerhut 2008)

3.3 Implications for women and for Programs and Organisations concerning HIV/AIDS

„Educar un hombre es educar un individuo, educar una mujer es educar una familia."[1]
Puebla, Mexico

As mentioned before, most HIV/AIDS prevention programs and NGOs focus on "vulnerable" groups, which somehow nearly always allude to women, and high-risk groups like *Injecting Drug Users* (IDUs), *Men who have Sex with Men* (MSM) and *Female Sex Workers* (FSWs). (UNAIDS 2008a: 213)

Concerning women, prevention-strategies focus on their vulnerability, which are given on the one hand through biological factors, and on the other hand through societal factors, as their often inferior position in society which translates into their sexual relationship. The result is, in regard to HIV/AIDS, a two to four times higher transmission from men to women than vice versa. (Red de Salud de Las Mujeres Latinoamericanas y del Caribe 2001: 32)

The still existing picture of the stereotypes, especially *Machismo* per se and the often secret sexual contacts between men are playing a grave role in the endangering of womens health, and further the health of their (unborn) children. (Galanti 2003: 180ff; Lampe 1999: 27; Marín 2003: 186; Moreno 2007: 340ff)

Due to the two Gender constructions *Marianismo* and *Machismo*, the sexuality of women and the sexuality of men are seen to be lived different. While women would learn to be monogamous, silent, passive and subjected to men and at their disposal, men on the contrary would experience that promiscuity, dominance and aggression concerning sexuality are the right behaviour. (Lampe 1999: 27)

As a womens body is perceived as belonging to others for providing pleasure, offering care and giving life without much consideration for her own, the position to influence the sexual behaviour of their partner of husband is not the best. (Red de Salud de Las Mujeres Latinoamericanas y del Caribe 2001: 32)

This complicated and still complicates the promotion of condoms. Gracia Violeta, a 27 year old Bolivian refered to this problem: "How are you going to convince a man to put on a condom without him hitting you, thinking you have a boyfriend on your side? How can a woman manage that" (World Vision International 2004: 109) This reaction of men also results because of the former promotion campaigns for condoms, which were adressing primarily

---

[1] "Education of a man is education of an individual, education of a woman is education of a family."

FSWs. Mostly, if women dare to negotiate safer-sex and using a condom, they are exposed to violence, which includes also sexual violence. (Lampe 1999: 27)

One possibility to, not really bypass this problem, but at least to widen the womens more independent scope of action and security for themselves, could be the femidom, or female condom.

In June 2008, the medical journal The Lancet Infectious Diseases dedicated an article to the female condomand its importance, wherein it is adverted to its underusage as prevention tool, against unwanted pregnancy as well as against sexually transmitted diseases (STDs) including HIV. Although the female condom was launched on the global markets over a decade ago, it accounts for just 0-2% of total condom supply. It is still the only female-initiated intervention for prevention, while other "new" men-orientated intervetions, like the male circumsission are receiving greater attention, (financial) support and promotion.

In Latin America, the only country that has successfully promoted the female condom, is Brazil. As a result, many women from other countries, who could benefit, can't access it or probably haven't heard of it. (The Lancet Infectious Diseases 2008: 343)

Of course, there are critics of the female condom, but as we seek to reduce the prevalence of STDs and especially HIV, I think it demands to use everything we have got in our tool kit, particularly if it is the only intervention for women to initiate protection.

If we take a look at the programs and NGOs concerning HIV/AIDS, the implications resulting from the two Gender concepts are, that the main approach should aim for the "empowerment of women". This is seen as vital to reversing the epidemic. (Lampe 1999: 20; Türmen 2003: 416ff)

"Empowerment of women" focuses on offering "tools" to expand their scope of action. Eighter gender considerations are incorporated into HIV education programs, or HIV/AIDS topics are incorporated in already existing organisations and programs, which were specialized in helping women to cope or overcome their cultural and societal determinated situation, through showing them and supporting ways of more (economic) independecy. (Lampe 1999: 19f; Türmen 2003: 417)

Their aims and topics are also to encourage discussion of the ways in which boys and girls are brought up and expected to behave, to challenge concepts of masculinity and femininity, based on inequality and aggressive and passive stereotypes; furthermore to teach female assertiveness in relationships and skills to negotiate safer-sex due to HIV/AIDS and other STDs, as well as to fight stigma. Equally, concerning the possible transmission of the disease

7

but also family-planning, the usage of contraceptives is taught. Finally, these programs seek also to challenge the norms about female sexuality, which is perceived to live passive, generous and obedient - resulting from the Gender constructions. (Lampe 1999: 20; Türmen 2003: 417) These aims and topics are seen as essential to tackle the increasing HIV/AIDS prevanlence in women.

All that appears and sounds really good, and encourages an optimistic feeling because it seems to cover nearly everything - at first sight. If one steps back a little bit, to watch the whole picture, what becomes visuable and perceived, is the burden for women underneath.
It is about time to ask: Where, in what way and to what extent is the (hetero- and/or hidden bisexual) male population involved?

Already in the 1990s this problem was acknowledged, as Birgit Lampe (1999: 20) pointed out: "Die Programme richten sich "Grundsätzlich an Frauen ohne Männer auszuschließen.'"[2] Nevertheless, that time two thirds of organisations concerning HIV/AIDS and Gender, which cooperated with her in her research, were working exclusively with women. She also refers to the intention of many NGOs, to increase the involvement of heterosexual men and even to concipate special programs for them, as women shouldn`t be stuck in their traditional role, being resposible and the "guarantress" for family-health, through letting them carry the liability for comunicationabout HIV/AIDS and "safer-sex" further on.
Being optimistic because of this important notice, one may be disapointed five years later, having to read, that there is still seen "the need to empower them (ann.:*the women*) to discuss with their partners (...) and to raise awareness on their contraceptive choices in a way to protect their own health, their partner`s health and even their unborn offspring`s health." (Cerqueira 2004: 2004)
Education and access to information about HIV/AIDS and its prevention is unquestionable life-saving, but adressing just one party (of two) will never bring the results that could be possible, if both parties would be approached. I think, likewise, to overcome the harmful and sometimes life-threatening outcomes of Gender constructions as well as Gender inequalities and inequaties, men and women should be in the picture about it.
Change needs time, but as the posibility to change is generally a part of the definition of culture per se, it will always happen. Sadly, the idea of changing behaviour of the female as well as of the (hetero- and/or hidden bisexual) male population, but just greatly adressing

---

[2] „The programs are addressing „ basically women without excluding men.'"

women – of course, also with good concepts but somehow bad in accomplishing - has up to now built up a wall, a barrier, around the hetero- and/or bisexual man, due to his exclusion from discussions and approaching.

Finally, I want to point out that I don`t see myself actually speaking against "empowerment of women", as equality of all Genders should exist, but I think it is time to split the burden intailed on women by one`s peer, concerning HIV/AIDS.

4. Conclusio

In my paper I provided an insight into the situation of women in Latin America concerning the disease.

Reviewing the "feminization" of HIV/AIDS, I reflected the impacts of the two major Gender constructing concepts of Latin America, *Machismo* and *Marianismo*, on (the development of) programs and organisations concerning the epidemic, and following, on women.

What has been showen is that *Machismo* and *Marianismo* are still seen to have consequences on the life situation of the female population, and can be life-threatening concerning the epidemic. Nevertheless, I think we should step away from making Gender constructions, and especially *Machismo* and the risky manly, the *Macho* behaviour responsible for the transmission of HIV/AIDS, but concentrating just on "vulnerable" women to stop it. I don`t think adressing nearly exclusive women, in respect of a heterosexual relationship, is and will be able to impede the increase of infections with the HI-virus. Also, it is important to unburden women, to release their resposibility to be the provider of health for the whole family, including the husband, as has been pointed out already ten years ago.

My conclusion is, due to given approaches to decrease the prevalence of the epidemic in Latin America, that it is time look for a proper way to reach also the male population, as well as to concentrate on (financial) support, promotion and provision of intervention for women to initiate protection, like the femidom or female condom, which I see as putting women into a more active position.

"Feminization of HIV/AIDS" today, in Latin America as well as everywhere else, shouldn`t be seen to adress and to deal with only the female population, as literature on Gender does not just focus on women. Of course, it is important to make Gender-inequaties and inequalities visible, may they be because of cultural, societal or biological factors, but to improve the life situation of women concerning HIV/AIDS, which would also affect their children, it is time to involve all parties and tobreak down the wall, the barrier around the (hetero- and/or hidden bisexual) male population.

References

CERQUEIRA, Ana Teresa de Abreu Ramos et al.
2004   Medidas contraceptivas e de proteção da transmissão do HIV
                        por mulheres com HIV/Aids. In: Revista de Saúde Pública,
                        2004, Vol. 38, No. 2, April: 194-200.

CHANT, Sylvia
2003   Introduction. Gender in a Changing Continent. In: Chant,
                        Sylvia/Craske, Nikki (Ed.): Gender in Latin America. London:
                        1-18.

GALANTI, Geri-Ann
2003   The Hispanic family and male-female relationships. An
                        overview. In: Journal of Transcultural Nursing, 2003, Vol. 14,
                        No. 3, July: 180-185.

LAMPE, Birgit
1999   Die Bedeutung von "Gender" in lateinamerikanischen
                        HIV/AIDS-Programmen. Eine Befragung von Nicht-
                        Regierungsorganisationen. Berlin.

MARÍN, Barbara Vanoss
2003   HIV Prevention in the Hispanic Community. Sex, Culture, and
                        Empowerment. In: Journal of Transcultural Nursing, 2003, Vol.
                        14, No. 3, July: 186-192.

MELHUUS, Marit/STOLEN, Kristi Anne
1996   Machos, Mistresses, Madonnas. Contesting the Power of Latin
                        American Gender Imagery. London, New York.

MORENO, Claudia L
2007   The Relationship Between Culture, Gender, Structural Factors,
                        Abuse, Trauma, and HIV/AIDS for Latinas. In: Qualitative
                        Health Research, 2007, Vol. 17, No. 3, March: 340-352.

Red de Salud de Las Mujeres Latinoamericanas y del Caribe
2001   AIDS in Latin America and the Caribbean. More female,
                        younger and poorer. / SIDA en América Latina y el Caribe. Más
                        femenino, más joven y más pobre. In: In: LOLA press, may
                        2001 – oct. 2001, No. 15: 30-33.

STEVENS, Evelyn
1973   Marianismo. The Other Face of Machism in Latin America. In:
                        Pescatelo, Ann (Ed.): Female and Male in Latin America,
                        Pittsburgh 1973.

THE LANCET Infectious Diseases
2008   The female condom. Still an underused prevention tool. In: The
                                 Lancet Infectious Diseases, 2008, Vol. 8, June: 343.

TÜRMEN, T.
2003   Gender   and   HIV/AIDS.   In: International   Journal   of
                                 Gynaecology and Obstetrics, 2003, Vol. 82, No. 3, Sept.: 411-
                                 418.

UNAIDS
2007   AIDS Epidemic Update 2007.
                                 http://data.unaids.org/pub/EPISlides/2007/2007_epiupdate_en.p
                                 df (19.02.2009)

UNAIDS
2008   HIV and AIDS Estimates and Data 2007 and 2001. In: 2008
                                 Report on the Global AIDS Epidemic: 211-234.
                                 http://viewer.zmags.com/publication/ad3eab7c#/ad3eab7c/6
                                 (19.02.2009)

World Vision International
2004   HIV-Positive Lives in latin america and the caribbean. Myths,
                                 realities, responses.
                                 http://www.childrights.org/PolicyAdvocacy/pahome2.5.nsf/
                                 cractionnews/1B92B42B641AF38688256F62001D3C9E/$file/
                                 HIV_Positive_lives.pdf (20.02.2009, 12:30)

ZUCKERHUT, Patricia
2008   Getauschte Sexualität, hybride Identität - Zur
                                 Geschlechterforschung Lateinamerikas. Machismus und
                                 Marianismus. Wien, NIG, Kultur-und Sozialanthropologie, HS
                                 C, 23.10.2008, 17-19 Uhr.